Dear Reader,

When Cristina Cuzzone was 9 years old, she was diagnosed with leukemia. After she underwent 6 weeks of chemotherapy, her health had not improved, so doctors recommended a bone marrow transplant. It was a scary time for Cristina and her family. They didn't know anyone who had been through a transplant and weren't sure what to expect. But Cristina bravely endured her treatment.

A few years later, Cristina spoke up: "There should be a book for kids that explains all about transplants!" she said. We agreed, and this book is the result of Cristina's inspiration. In it, you'll learn what transplants are, how they are done, what your treatment will feel like, and ways to cope during difficult times. Throughout the book, Cristina is your special guide. She offers helpful tips and explains what she was thinking and feeling during each stage of her treatment.

This book will remind you that you're not alone. Each year, more than 2,000 kids in the U.S. get bone marrow transplants. Many of them have also shared their advice and experiences in these pages, hoping to make your transplant easier for you.

You can read this book from beginning to end or flip through it and just read pages on certain topics. We hope it will answer your questions and help you feel more comfortable during your transplant. Best wishes for a smooth journey through your treatment and a bright future ahead!

Your friends at Astellas

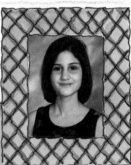

Cristina, age 13
4 years after transplant

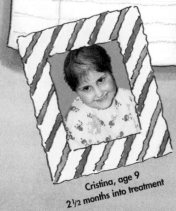

Cristina, age 9
2½ months into treatment

Cristina Cuzzone

Table of Contents

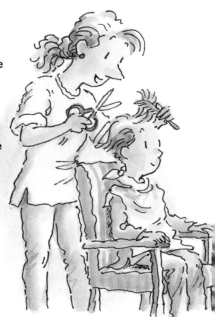

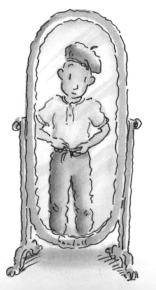

After Your Transplant

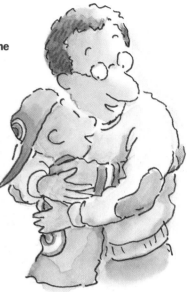

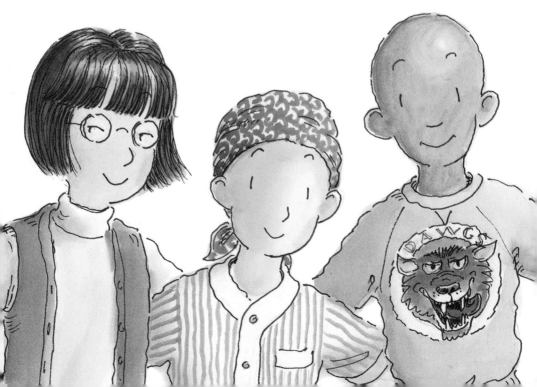

Getting the News

A Flood of Feelings

A bone marrow transplant is a complicated procedure. The more you understand about your treatment, though, the less stressful it will probably be. This book will explain what you can expect during each phase of your transplant and teach you ways to help yourself feel better.

When you first learned you needed a transplant, you may have felt **afraid.** Or you might have been **confused** about what lay ahead. You may have been **angry** if you've undergone other difficult treatment that didn't cure your disease. Or maybe you felt **shocked,** and unable to think. These are all normal reactions. In fact, you may have felt several of these emotions at the same time.

"I didn't understand the terms the doctors used, but I didn't worry—I knew the transplant was only going to make me better," Cristina says. "I knew eventually I'd understand. They explained it all to me again later."

Talking about It

Bone marrow transplants can be overwhelming—there's so much to learn about the treatment you'll be receiving. You and your family might feel worried or frustrated at times. It's OK to cry. It's also OK if you don't want to hear details about your treatment or discuss your transplant right away. When you *are* ready, though, sharing your feelings with family members, friends, or hospital caregivers can help. Talking about your fears and hopes can strengthen your relationships, which will support you through the challenges to come.

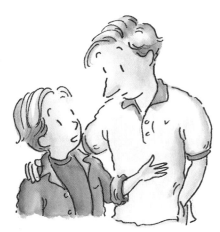

The Road to Recovery

The journey ahead of you will not be easy, but remember: other kids have gone down this road before you and say that it's worth it. You can help yourself get well by trying to keep a positive attitude. That doesn't mean you have to be cheerful or brave all the time—after all, having a transplant stinks! Just remember that every part of your treatment is necessary to make you better.

Take one day at a time. Don't worry about what will happen a few weeks or months from now. Control the things you can, and leave the rest to your doctors and nurses. Whenever possible, laugh and smile. Set goals for yourself, both in the hospital and beyond. Talk about your dreams and plans for your future. If you keep your hopes high, your body will have more energy to heal itself.

Mixed Emotions

These kids explain how they felt when they got the news.

 "I was angry and really upset because I had gone through so much already and it wasn't working. But if you have cancer, you try anything."

Nathan S.
Age 15, 3 1/2 years after transplant

 "I really didn't understand it all, but I knew my mom and dad were scared, so that scared me."

Audra B.
Age 9, 3 years after transplant

 "I was excited because I knew I could get better by getting someone else's bone marrow."

Katie E.
Age 12, 2 years after transplant

Bone Marrow Basics

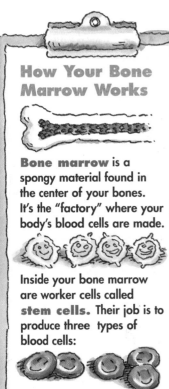
What is a BMT?

Bone marrow transplants, or "BMTs," are performed to treat many types of cancer and other diseases. During a BMT, healthy bone marrow cells—specifically, *stem cells*—are transplanted into a person who has diseased or damaged marrow. (That's why BMTs are also called "stem cell transplants," or "SCTs.")

Why do I need one?

Blood Diseases: Many kids who need a BMT or SCT have bone marrow that isn't working properly. Kids with leukemia—like Cristina—have bone marrow that is overproducing abnormal white blood cells. The abnormal cells crowd out the normal cells and keep them from doing their job. Kids with other blood diseases may have marrow that doesn't produce *enough* blood cells. A transplant can help correct these kinds of diseases by replacing the patient's unhealthy bone marrow cells with healthy cells that work properly. The healthy stem cells build a new bone marrow factory where healthy blood cells are then produced.

Solid Tumor Cancers: Some kids have a cancerous tumor in their body that's especially hard to get rid of. When this happens, doctors use *very* high doses of chemotherapy and sometimes also radiation therapy to make the tumor go away. Unfortunately, this high-dose treatment also damages the healthy cells in the patient's bone marrow. To help the patient rebuild his or her bone marrow factory, doctors remove some of the patient's marrow or stem cells to save. Then after the radiation or chemotherapy treatment is over, they give the saved stem cells back to the patient as a bone marrow "rescue."

Where will the healthy stem cells come from?

Your new stem cells will be donated by someone whose marrow type closely matches your own. Family members will be tested to see whether their marrow is a good match. If not, the hospital will look for a donor who is not related to you. Sometimes patients can donate stem cells back to themselves. Your doctor will let you know whether this is possible. If not, finding a donor could take months. As you wait, doctors will treat your illness the best they can. During this time, try to build your strength through a healthy diet and exercise. (Pages 24-25 explain more about marrow matching and cell collection.)

How are the new stem cells transplanted?

You'll receive the donated stem cells through an IV. They'll travel through your bloodstream to the space in the center of your bones. There, they'll set up their factory and start producing healthy new blood cells. (See pages 26-27 to read more about the transplant experience.)

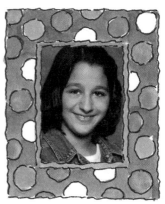

"In the beginning, I didn't want to know anything about my treatment. But later, I wanted to know everything that was going to happen—no secrets. When I know what's going on, I'm not as scared."

Brittany P.
Age 12, 3 years after transplant

About one-third of all BMT patients will have a sibling whose bone marrow is a good match.

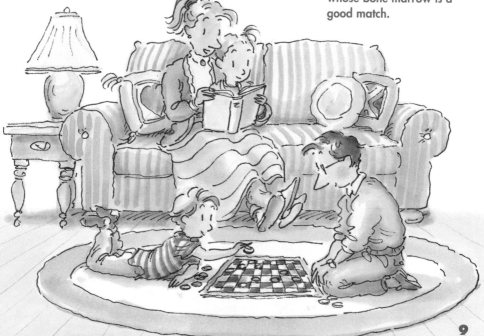

Hospital Questions

For the next several months, your transplant doctors and nurses will be providing you with special care. You'll spend some of that time in the hospital. The more prepared you are for your stay, the more comfortable you'll be. Here are answers to some common questions kids have about their hospital stay. These pages will help you know what to expect *before* you go.

What will happen when I arrive?

Once you're admitted, you'll be taken on a tour of the transplant unit to see how the equipment works and to meet the people who will be involved with your treatment. They'll explain procedures and tell you some of the things you can expect.

How long will I be there?

Usually patients spend one or more months in the hospital, but every patient's situation is different. How quickly you can be discharged depends on how quickly your bone marrow and body recover from the transplant.

Will I be able to see my family?

Once your treatment has begun and your risk of infection becomes greater, you may only be allowed to have one or two family visitors. Some hospitals permit a parent to stay in your room with you, especially if the hospital is far from your home.

Who are all these people?

The members of your treatment team are experts in BMTs and SCTs. Besides the doctors and nurses who specialize in transplants, you'll probably also work with the following people.

Transplant coordinator: explains special procedures and treatment to you throughout your stay.

Dietician or nutritionist: meets with you to create menus based on foods that you like and that will aid your recovery.

Child-life specialist: helps you and your family adjust to hospital life.

Hospital dentist: examines your mouth, teeth, and gums throughout your transplant and treats any problems.

Radiation technician: uses radiation to prepare your body for the transplant.

Phlebotomist: collects blood samples for testing.

Physical therapist: helps you exercise and stay fit while you're in the hospital.

Will I have tests?

Doctors may want you to have the following tests to make sure you're as healthy as possible. (Any infections—no matter how small—must be treated and eliminated before the transplant can be done.) Doctors will also compare the tests done before and after your transplant to see how your body may have changed due to your treatment.

Chest x-ray: to check your lungs for pneumonia.

EKG (electrocardiogram): to look at your heart rhythm.

Sample "cultures": taken of throat, urine, stool, and nose to check for infections.

Blood draws: to check your blood-cell counts.

Get Comfortable!

In some hospitals, you'll stay in a special germ-free room from the time you're admitted until you're discharged. In others, you'll move into a new room after your transplant. Either way, you'll probably feel more at home if you fix up your space to **make it yours.** Bring things from home to help you **pass the time** and **make yourself comfortable.**

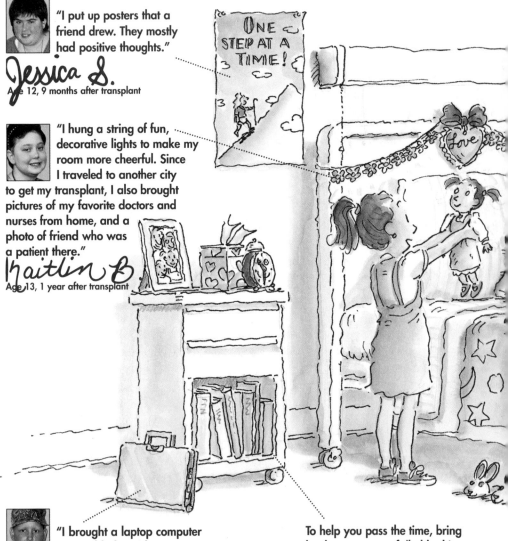

"I put up posters that a friend drew. They mostly had positive thoughts."

Jessica S.
Age 12, 9 months after transplant

"I hung a string of fun, decorative lights to make my room more cheerful. Since I traveled to another city to get my transplant, I also brought pictures of my favorite doctors and nurses from home, and a photo of friend who was a patient there."

Kaitlin B.
Age 13, 1 year after transplant

ONE STEP AT A TIME!

"I brought a laptop computer so I could play video games and go on the internet."

Keith H.
Age 14, 1 month after transplant

To help you pass the time, bring books, games, craft/hobby kits, stationery, your address book, videotapes, CDs or audiotapes, and a Walkman or boom box.

"The first thing doctors wanted me to do was to make the room look the way I wanted it to. I put up pictures of my family and made a big collage on the wall of all the cards I got," says Cristina.

To make your hospital stay more comfortable, bring loose-fitting clothes, pajamas, slippers, a robe, and a quilt or pillow from your bed at home.

"I brought my stuffed animals and my pillow from Camp Sunshine—a camp for kids with cancer."

MARQUES M.

Age 14, 6 weeks after transplant

Important!

Leave live plants and flowers at home—your room must be kept sterile. (Plants may carry fungi, molds, or bacteria that could cause serious infections.) Check to see if your hospital has any other restrictions.

Preparing Your Body

Your Central Line

During your transplant, you'll be given lots of injected medicines, blood transfusions, and other IV fluids like liquid nutrients. You'll also need to have blood samples drawn and checked every day. So that these procedures can be done painlessly, your doctor will give you a *central line*—a tube that's surgically placed in your chest. It will connect to a large vein and enable your transplant team to care for you without poking you with needles several times a day.

Chemotherapy

Before you're given your new stem cells, doctors need to prepare your body for them. About a week before your transplant, you'll begin receiving chemotherapy. You may have had chemotherapy before, but this time the doses of medicine will be *much* stronger. The chemotherapy not only has to kill any cancer cells still in your body (if you have cancer), it also has to destroy your bone marrow cells so they won't fight off the new donated cells once they're transplanted. (Chemotherapy can sometimes have uncomfortable side effects. See pages 16-18 for coping suggestions.)

The nurse will change your central line's dressing every day. The area may feel a little tender at first, but any discomfort will go away in a day or two.

Radiation Therapy

In addition to chemotherapy, you may also receive radiation therapy to prepare your body for your transplant. Powerful x-rays will be aimed at your body to help destroy your bone marrow and any cancer cells. The x-rays are the same kind used to see a broken bone, but they're given in much higher doses.

How radiation is given: Before your treatment, the technician will measure your body and mark it with a pen. These marks help the technician guide the x-rays to the right places. Heavy lead pads, or "blocks," may be placed on parts of your body to protect sensitive organs. Because you must stay in one position without moving during the entire treatment, you may be given a medication to help you relax and remain still. Treatments usually last 10-15 minutes and may be given twice a day, several days in a row.

What it feels like: Getting radiation treatment is a lot like getting an x-ray: the machine makes a soft clicking sound and doesn't hurt. Some kids say their skin feels warm or tingly afterwards. You may feel tired and want to sleep when the treatment is over. In some hospitals, you can talk to the technician or family members through a speaker while receiving radiation. (Pages 19-21 give tips for making yourself more comfortable if you feel a little anxious during your treatment.)

A Well-Deserved Break

You will probably be given a break from all therapy on the day before your transplant. This gives your body time to recover and rid itself of some of the chemotherapy that could harm the new stem cells you'll be receiving.

Special Protection

After you receive chemotherapy/radiation therapy, your white blood cells will be destroyed. Germs that would normally not bother you can make you very sick at this stage. Cleanliness is especially important for you now.

To keep you safe from infection, doctors, nurses, and visitors may need to put on sanitary clothing such as hospital gowns, masks, and gloves before entering your room. Even more important, they'll have to scrub with special germ-killing soap. Hand-washing is the best method to control infection. In fact, many hospitals encourage kids to be the hand-washing police. Join the squad—ask everyone who comes into your room, including your doctors and nurses: "Have you washed your hands?"

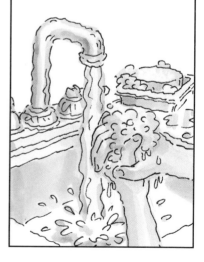

Side Effects, Head to Toe

Radiation therapy, chemotherapy, and other drugs used in transplants can cause unpleasant side effects. Most go away after treatment ends. You may experience **several**, a **few**, or **none** of the more common ones listed on these pages. Some side effects can be controlled by medications or by changing your diet or routine. Others can't be prevented, but knowing they are normal may help you worry less.

Hair Loss

Chemotherapy drugs destroy cancer cells and other cells that reproduce rapidly, like hair cells. With some people, hair just thins. With others, it falls out from a few sections of the scalp or completely—eyebrows and eyelashes included. Hair usually grows back within 3 to 6 months, sometimes a different shade or texture.

What you can do: If your hair is long, you may want to cut it short before your transplant so it's not such a drastic change if your hair starts to thin. Also, short hair is not as heavy as long hair, so hair that doesn't fall out will have a fuller look if it is shorter. (To read how other kids dealt with their thinning hair, turn to pages 30-32.)

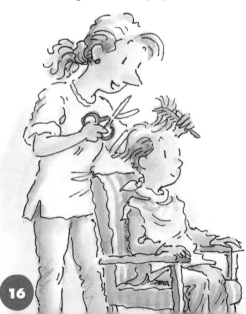

Fatigue

Many things can make you feel tired: your body is working overtime to heal itself; you're probably not sleeping as well as you did at home; you may not be eating enough due to nausea or loss of appetite; medicines that treat nausea and pain can cause drowsiness.

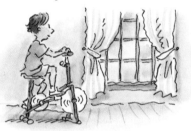

What you can do: Take naps during the day and eat well-balanced meals and snacks. Even though you're tired, it's important to exercise. Activity actually gives you energy and helps keep your body strong. On days when you have more energy, the physical therapist can make exercising fun. When you're feeling really drained, try at least to get up to bathe and clean your teeth.

Mood Changes

Treatment and medications may affect your personality, taking you on an emotional roller-coaster ride. You may feel normal one minute and upset the next.

What you can do: Talk to your doctor to find out if medications are causing your moodiness, and whether they can be adjusted.

Mouth Problems

Chemotherapy irritates the rapidly reproducing cells that line your mouth and throat. Sores may develop, making it hard to eat or swallow.

What you can do:

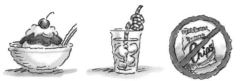

Eat cool, soft foods that are easy to chew and swallow (such as ice cream, cottage cheese, applesauce, and puddings).

Drink liquids through a straw. Suck on ice chips.

Avoid citrus fruit and juices, tomato sauces, spicy or salty foods (such as potato chips or pretzels), and rough or dry foods (such as crackers or toast).

Because your germ-fighting white blood cells were wiped out by chemotherapy, mouth sores can become infected. Also, because your platelet count is low, your gums may bleed after you eat or clean your teeth.

What you can do: Good oral care can actually *prevent* many mouth problems. Gently clean your teeth with a spongette and rinse with medicated mouthwashes several times a day. Rinsing often with saline water will also help remove food and bacteria.

Your taste buds may not work properly for several weeks after your transplant due to reduced saliva in your mouth or medications you're taking. Foods might taste different to you—they may have less taste or a bitter or metallic flavor.

What you can do: Once your treatment is over and your saliva glands and taste buds heal, food *will* taste good again. Until then, try increasing the seasoning in your foods. Drink water, eat hard candy, and chew gum to help make your mouth more moist.

The cleaner you keep your mouth, the better it will feel!

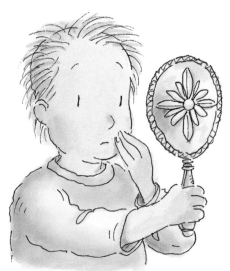

Changes in Body Appearance

Certain drugs may cause fluids to collect in your body, making your face, stomach, and legs swell.

What you can do: When your recovery is complete, your body will return to normal. In the meantime, your doctor may suggest you cut back on salty foods or give you medicine to help your body eliminate the extra fluid.

Nausea/Vomiting

Chemotherapy may upset your stomach. You may even begin to feel sick just thinking about your treatment before it begins.

What you can do: The nurse can give you medicine to lessen your nausea. It also helps to wear loose, comfortable clothing. Don't eat for a few hours before therapy. Instead, drink clear liquids like water, apple juice, or ginger ale. Later, when you feel you can eat, try dry, bland foods such as crackers or pretzels. Avoid warm foods, which can have strong smells that trigger nausea. Rest sitting up for an hour after meals.

Diarrhea

Chemotherapy irritates the cells that line your stomach and intestines. Your body isn't able to digest food as well, which can lead to diarrhea. Intestinal infections can also cause diarrhea, which may be severe.

What you can do: If it's hard to make it to the bathroom, ask for a portable toilet to be placed next to your bed. Nurses can give you medicated creams if you're sore from wiping. Avoid milk products, and greasy or spicy foods. Instead, eat bland foods low in fiber (noodles, white rice, or applesauce), and drink plenty of clear, room-temperature fluids. As your body heals from your transplant, you'll begin to feel better.

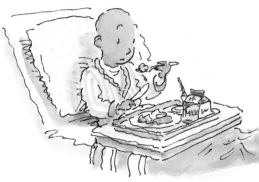

Inability to Eat

During the days of your transplant, a sore mouth and upset stomach may make eating just too difficult.

What you can do: If you just can't bring yourself to eat, don't worry. Your doctors will make sure you receive good nutrition through your IV or nasal tube. (It's important to keep your digestive system working if possible, though, so see pages 40-41 for more advice about eating.)

Mind over Body

Did you know your **mind** can actually make your **body** feel better? You can train your brain to help you **cope** with uncomfortable procedures or **boost** your mood on a bad day. To be successful, you must practice these mental tricks a few times before using them. Your child-life specialist or a nurse trained in these techniques can help you master them even better.

Relaxation

Worry or stress sometimes actually *causes* nausea and even pain. Here are a few techniques to relax your mind and help your body overcome pain, nausea, and other discomforts:

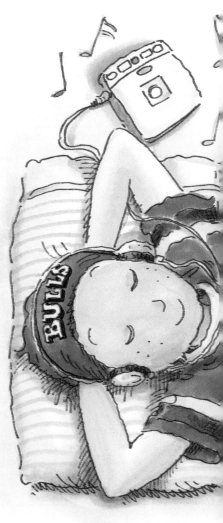

- **Get in a comfortable position. Breathe in deeply through your nose for a count of 3. Exhale slowly through your mouth, counting to 3. Each time you breathe out, let go of your tension or scary feelings. Visualize your pain or nausea leaving your body. Let it drain out of your head, shoulders, stomach, arms, and legs, down onto the floor, and away for good.**

- **Calming activities such as crossword puzzles, embroidery, and slow-paced computer games like solitaire slow your breathing and heart rate and help your muscles relax. Next time you feel tense, try a relaxing hobby to calm you down.**

Distraction

Give your mind something positive to focus on when you're uncomfortable; otherwise it may concentrate on negative feelings like fear or pain. To distract yourself during an unpleasant procedure, you can play mental games like this: try spelling the names of people in the room backwards. Simple things like talking, listening to music, or watching TV work, too.

"We'd do something different to keep my mind off things," Cristina says. "Like playing a new game— I'd have to really concentrate to learn how to play."

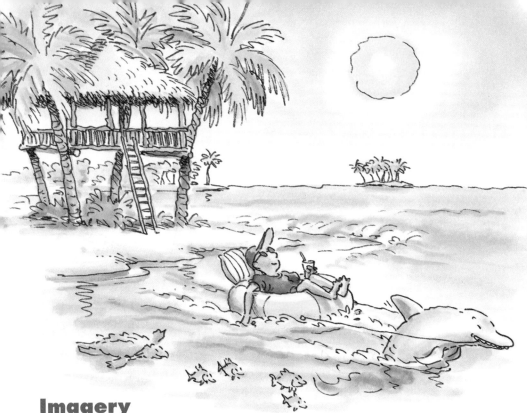

Imagery

Your mind can take you to a place far from the hospital and an uncomfortable procedure you're having. You can go anywhere you want! Here's how:

1 Find an object in the room and stare at it. Breathe deeply to relax your body. Then imagine a peaceful scene such as a sandy beach with waving palm trees, a clear blue sky, and bright sunshine.

2 Now imagine yourself on the beach. Use a variety of senses. **Feel** a warm breeze blowing. **Smell** the salty air. **See** sailboats in the distance. **Hear** seagulls crying and waves crashing. You can do anything you want here—build a sand castle, look for colorful seashells, or jump in the water and body surf. Let your mind be a movie screen, showing you pictures of things you enjoy. You might even write down your scene or record it on tape so you can listen to it later.

You can return to this place whenever you want or you can visit another. Here are some other relaxing scenes you might imagine:

- floating in a hot-air balloon among the clouds

- standing under a cool waterfall in a tropical forest

- lying under a tree in a field of colorful flowers

- watching the sunset with your dog

- walking with a friend on a moonlit night

You can also imagine yourself doing things you've enjoyed in the past—like relaxing with your family on a favorite vacation or holiday. Remember the good feelings, and your brain will relive the experience as if it's happening again.

Support from Others

Peace through prayer: Many people find strength in family, friends, and God. Some kids say that praying—by themselves, with a family member, or with a hospital chaplain—gives them hope and strength to fight their disease. If you belong to a youth group, praying with your leader or group members on the phone may also give you comfort.

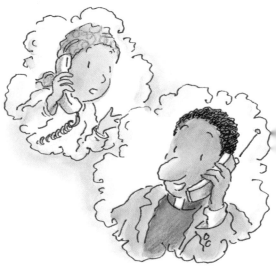

Connect through computers: If your hospital has the equipment, you may be able to e-mail family and friends or chat on-line with your classmates or other hospitalized kids across the country. You can visit **http://www.astellas.us** for a list of recommended networks, chat groups, and entertaining and helpful web sites.

Keep Spirits High

Here are some ways to keep a positive attitude, day in and day out.

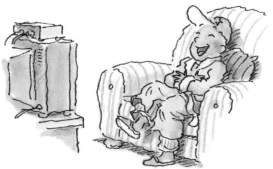

Just as a bad mood may make you feel sicker, **humor** helps heal. Ask family and friends to send you cards, letters, or videotapes that make you laugh.

Hang a **schedule** of your daily activities on your wall and ask your caregivers to respect your private times. This will help you get more done and give you more control over how you spend your days.

"We rented one movie that made me laugh so hard I didn't feel the bad effects of my medicine. I just felt so much better. Laughter definitely helps!

"My schedule made it easier for me to do the hard things. Instead of being tempted to skip things, I knew they'd help me get better. If it was on the schedule, it had to be done."

Zachary Z.
Age 15, 5 years after transplant

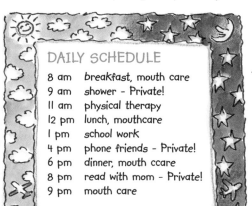

DAILY SCHEDULE

8 am	breakfast, mouth care
9 am	shower - Private!
11 am	physical therapy
12 pm	lunch, mouthcare
1 pm	school work
4 pm	phone friends - Private!
6 pm	dinner, mouth ccare
8 pm	read with mom - Private!
9 pm	mouth care

Tips for Talking

During your treatment, there may be days you wish you could run away from it all. You may feel angry when nurses or doctors perform unpleasant procedures or frightened when you don't know what to expect. Talking with your caregivers can help.

Discussion Dos and Don'ts

Here are some suggestions for how to talk about what worries you:

Don't be too frightened to ask questions about your treatment. Procedures are often less scary than you imagined. When you know what's ahead, you'll feel more control over the situation.

Do expect truthful answers. You may not want to hear that a procedure is going to hurt, but being surprised is usually worse.

Don't be afraid to ask the same question more than once, or that your questions will sound dumb. Most of us don't know much about how our bodies work. Doctors and nurses will be glad you're interested and want to help you learn more.

Do expect clear explanations about your treatment. To help you get comfortable with new equipment, doctors or nurses may demonstrate or let you try a new procedure on a doll before it's done to you.

Don't worry that your questions take up too much of your doctor's time. It's your body, and you have a right to learn what's going on. If you're asleep or in the bathroom when your doctor stops by, see if he or she can come back when you can talk.

Do write down your questions so you'll remember them, and jot down the answers when you get them. If you're feeling too sick to ask your questions, have a family member ask and write the answers for you. Below are some questions you may have.

1. What will happen?
2. Where will it happen?
3. Who will be there?
4. What equipment will be used, and what does it do?
5. What will it feel like when it is used?
6. How often will I need to have this done?

"If my nurses were giving me a medicine that would make me feel bad, they'd tell me," Cristina says. "And when they said it *wasn't* going to hurt, I could relax because I knew they were telling the truth."

Participation Pointers

Did you know you can sometimes help make decisions about your treatment? Doctors or nurses may be able to make a procedure more comfortable if they know how you feel. Here are some ways to get more involved in your care:

- If you feel better when a parent is with you for a procedure—to hold your hand or talk to you—ask what treatment they may be able to stay with you for.

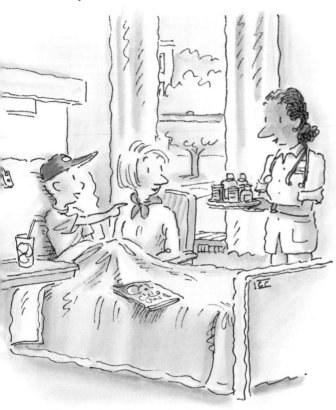

- You may be able to make choices about some of your routines, such as which medication to take first or what position you want to be in for procedures. Let your doctors and nurses know if you have a request.

- You'll be working with your treatment team for a long time—make friends with them. Ask them about themselves: what they like to do for fun, or what their favorite kind of music is. Good friends make good teammates!

Cristina's Story

Learn More, Fear Less!

Whenever Cristina had to undergo a new procedure, her caregivers made it like a science project. The doctors showed Cristina her x-rays and explained them to her. Technicians let her look at her blood samples under a microscope to see how her cells were doing. And when she had stomach problems that needed to be checked, doctors used a special camera o take internal pictures, then showed the photos to Cristina. Learning about all these things made new procedures less scary for Cristina.

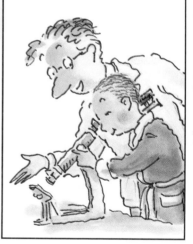

The Harvest

The procedure to **collect** the donated bone marrow or stem **cells** is called the *harvest*. Before the harvest can take place, a **donor** must be found. If tests show that your brother or sister can be your donor, you may want to share these pages with him or her.

Why Marrow Must Match

Only cells that are very similar to your own can be used for your transplant. If your marrow type did not match your donor's, the transplanted cells would notice that your body's cells were different, and attack them.

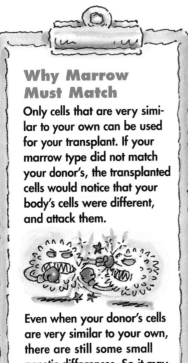

Even when your donor's cells are very similar to your own, there are still some small genetic differences. So it may take time for your body's cells and the transplanted cells to learn to work together.

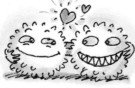

If you're donating cells back to yourself, your recovery will probably be quicker. The transplanted cells and your body's cells won't fight at all because they'll be old friends.

Finding a Donor

Your donor will be one of the following people:

- yourself
- a sibling or other family member
- someone not related to you

Whether or not you'll be able to donate your own stem cells depends on the type of disease you have and your current condition. Your doctor will let you know if you can be your own donor.

If you have a sibling, there's a 25 percent chance that his or her bone marrow type will match yours. An identical twin's marrow will match yours exactly. Unfortunately, it's likely that none of your family members will have matching bone marrow. Then an unrelated donor must be found. A search for a suitable donor will be carried out in the U.S. and even foreign countries.

Collecting Stem Cells

The stem cells you'll receive will be collected from one of three places:

- a person's bone marrow—the largest amount is found in the hip bones
- blood that's circulating through a person's body—these stem cells are called *peripheral* (pe-RIF-er-al) stem cells
- the umbilical cord of a newborn baby—full of stem cells

A Donor's Experience

Bone marrow donor: The donor enters the hospital on the day of, or day before, your transplant. He or she sleeps through the harvest and doesn't feel anything during it. Doctors use a needle to remove a small amount of marrow from the donor's hip bones. The donor leaves the hospital later that day or the next and may feel a little sore in the hips, as if he or she fell while roller-blading.

Peripheral stem cell donor: The donor is hooked up to an *apheresis* (ay-fur-EE-sis) machine which draws blood from one arm, filters it to collect stem cells, then returns the leftover blood to the other arm. The procedure is painless but takes several hours and may be repeated a few times before your transplant to get enough cells. The cells are frozen until the day of your transplant.

Umbilical cord donor: After a baby is born, the umbilical cord is disconnected. Stem cells inside the cord are collected and stored until they're ready to be used by someone like you.

Donating to yourself: Your bone marrow stem cell harvest will take place before your chemotherapy/radiation therapy since these treatments destroy the cells in your marrow.

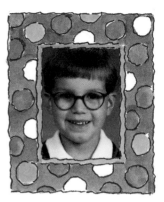

"I wrote a letter to my donor to thank him for giving me his bone marrow. I call him my 'Blood Brother.' We still stay in touch."

chris S.
Age 6 1/2, 4 years after transplant

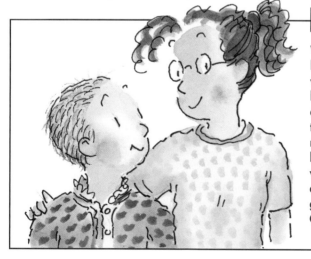

Cristina's Story

When Cristina found out that her half-sister Antonia's marrow was a good match, she was very happy. But Cristina also felt bad about putting Antonia through the harvest. Antonia said, "You're my sister—you don't have to feel bad." Antonia was a little nervous about the harvest, but she also felt she had a very special gift to give—the chance to help Cristina become healthy again.

The Transplant

It may surprise you that kids often say their bone marrow transplant or rescue is **anticlimactic**—not that big an event compared to other procedures they've had. Maybe that's because BMTs and SCTs aren't surgeries. They're **infusions** (slow injections), similar to blood transfusions. Here's what to **expect** on your transplant day and beyond.

Receiving Your Cells

On the day of your transplant, the donated stem cells will be given to you through your central line. It takes close to an hour for the cells to drip from their IV bag into your bloodstream. You'll feel no pain and can talk to family members, watch TV, or just rest. You'll be given medications before the transplant to prevent serious reactions from occurring. Nurses and doctors will watch you closely to treat any reactions you may have.

How Your Body Responds

Reactions during transplants are not very common. Taking deep breaths might cause you to cough due to tiny particles in the donated marrow moving through your lungs' blood vessels. Sometimes patients get chills, a mild fever, or a skin rash. Your urine may also turn pink or red for a few days, which is normal—your body's just getting rid of extra red blood cells that may have been mixed in with the stem cells.

If you're receiving marrow or stem cells that were frozen (because you donated them earlier or they were shipped from another state or country), you may notice a smell or a taste similar to garlic. This is a common side effect. It's caused by the chemical that the stem cells were stored in to keep them healthy for you. The taste or odor lasts a day or two. Your nurse can give you medicine if it makes you feel nauseous.

T-Day Thoughts

Kids remember their transplant day in different ways.

"My brother was my donor. Now my family celebrates my transplant day as a holiday. We call it 'Togetherness Day.' Since that day, my brother and I will always be together—no matter what."

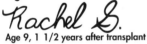

Age 9, 1 1/2 years after transplant

"When I got my cells, the taste in my mouth was bad. I ate mint candy to cover it up. The candy really helped."

Gabriel G.

Age 10, 8 months after transplant

The Wait

Once the donated cells have dripped into your bloodstream, they'll make their way to their new home in the center of your bones. Then the waiting begins. On average, it takes about 14 to 30 days for your new marrow to *engraft*, or begin producing new blood cells. This must happen before you can leave the hospital. Doctors will test your blood every day to check your progress.

It may seem like it takes forever for your new marrow to engraft. You may not notice much change in the way you feel from day to day—you might take a small step forward or backward or have no change at all. The slow recovery pace can be frustrating. Though it's important to have goals for your recovery, try to take one day at a time, and not focus *too* far into the future. When you do reach your recovery goals, celebrate!

Day 0, and Beyond

From this point on, your days will probably be referred to by numbers. The day of your transplant is considered Day 0. Although your marrow may engraft as soon as Day 14, it's not unusual for this to happen *after* Day 30. You may stay in the hospital even longer if you experience complications.

The first 100 days—or 3 months—after your transplant are the most critical because it takes at least that long for your bone marrow to build its *immune* (infection-fighting) system. During this time you're at the highest risk for complications that will affect your recovery. (To read about the most common transplant complications, turn the page.)

Possible Complications

Infection

Your bone marrow was destroyed by chemotherapy/radiation. Until your new marrow is able to produce infection-fighting white blood cells, your body won't be able to defend itself against germs. Infection can be the most serious complication right after your transplant.

■ You may begin protective isolation if you haven't already. Your contact with people will be limited to your doctors, nurses, and a few visitors.

■ Fevers are a sign of infection. They are very common. If you develop one, you'll be given antibiotics to fight the infection.

■ Bathe daily to help remove germs from your skin. Hand-washing is still the best way to prevent infection.

■ Good oral care will keep mouth sores from becoming infected.

■ Fresh fruits and vegetables will be eliminated from your diet since they may contain bacteria. All your food must be thoroughly cooked.

If you've been hospitalized for a long time and are feeling restless, you may be able to go for walks in the halls at night. It's less crowded then, so exposure to germs is less likely.

Most complications are due to **treatment** you received before transplant or drugs given to prevent side effects. Here are some problems that **delay** recovery and what you may be able to do to **prevent** them.

Acute GVHD

If you received your own marrow or cells donated by an identical twin, you won't have to worry about this complication. But if your cells were donated by another person, there's a chance you'll experience some form of GVHD, or "graft-versus-host disease." GVHD occurs when the donated cells attack your body cells because they are different. The donor cells usually target the skin, liver, and intestines. You may develop a rash, stomach pains, vomiting, diarrhea, or jaundice—yellow skin or eyes.

■ Medications will be given to stop the donated cells' attack. But these drugs also prevent your body from fighting off other intruders like germs, so your infection risk will be greater.

Bleeding

Since you received high doses of chemotherapy/radiation, your body's platelet count is low. Until your new marrow is able to produce more platelets, you can bleed easily.

■ You'll get platelet transfusions to help your blood clot.
■ Your nose may feel itchy or dry, but resist the urge to touch it. If you must blow it, do so gently—it will bleed easily and the flow may be hard to stop.
■ Don't worry if you see blood in your urine, stool, or vomit. That's just a sign you need another platelet transfusion.

Graft Failure

Most often, stem cells engraft and start to make new blood for you.

■ If there is a problem and they don't engraft, you may receive another infusion of cells.

Going to the ICU

If you need more—or different—care than the BMT unit can provide, you'll go to the ICU (Intensive Care Unit). It's in a different area of the hospital with a different team of caregivers.

■ This move will make you better faster. The ICU and BMT doctors will work together to help you recover and return you to the BMT unit as soon as you're able.

Physical Changes

The inside of your body has been going through many changes during your treatment. You're probably experiencing changes on the outside as well. For some kids, **hair** loss or **weight** loss (or unwanted gains) are especially upsetting. Here are some suggestions for what you can do to **look good** and **feel better** at this time.

Hip Headgear

Even if you expect your appearance to change as a result of your treatment, it can still be a shock when this actually happens. Give yourself time to adjust to the changes. It may not be easy at first, but remember: although these changes will be with you for a while, they probably won't last forever.

Hair loss is often the most difficult body change to accept. Whether you wear a head covering is up to you. Many kids experiment with different looks to find what's most comfortable for them. Here are some you may want to try.

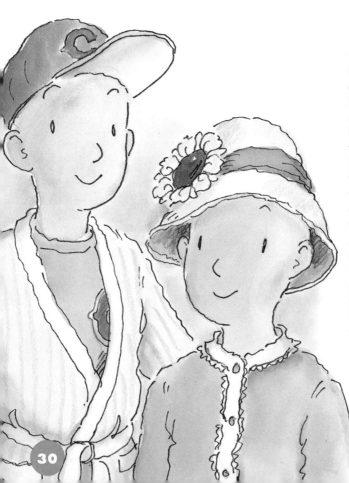

Caps or Hats

Hair takes up space, so hats or caps that you wore before you lost your hair may be too big now. If you buy a new hat, keep in mind that your hair won't be there to cushion your head, so check the hat's inside for scratchy seams. Hats made from natural fibers like cotton are most comfortable. You may want to have a few different styles for different occasions: dress, play, sleeping (without hair, your head gets cold), and protection outdoors (make sure the hat covers your entire hairline—down the back of your head).

Wigs

If you want to get a wig, it will help to take photos of your former hair style from the front, side, and back. Also take a small sample of your hair to the store if you want the wig's color to match your own—or you might want to take this opportunity to try a different hair color or style. If possible, have the wig cut and styled while you're wearing it.

When you wear a wig, air can't reach your scalp. Your head may perspire, making your scalp itch or feel hot. If this happens, try wearing a small cloth cap under the wig to absorb the perspiration.

Scarves and Bandannas

You can learn one tying technique and change fabrics to suit different occasions.

To tie a basic bandanna: fold a bandanna or square scarf in half to make a triangle.

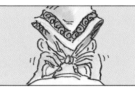

Place the scarf on your head with the point of the triangle in back, then tie the two ends at the back of your neck.

For a different look, try wearing the knot on the side, or add a hat over the scarf.

Going Natural

You may feel best without any head covering at all. That's fine, but when you're outside you'll still need some kind of protection. Hair keeps your body from losing heat, so in colder weather pull on a hat or head scarf to keep you warm. Your hair also protects your scalp from the sun's rays (which can be harmful even on cloudy days), so wear a hat and use a sunscreen with an SPF (sun protection factor) of at least 15. This is especially important if you are at risk for GVHD because the sun can activate GVHD or make it worse.

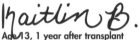

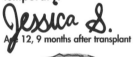
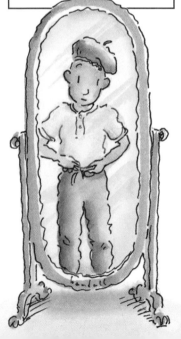

A Weighty Issue

Certain medications that are part of your treatment can cause your body to hold onto extra fluids, making it swell. Other drugs may make you hungrier than normal, so you eat more and put on extra pounds. Or, you may have the opposite problem—a lack of appetite that causes you to lose weight and not look yourself.

Although your appetite and body size should return to normal once your treatment is over, until then you may worry about your appearance. If your clothes no longer fit, here are some suggestions for keeping you comfortably in style:

■ Loose shirts or drawstring pants can adjust to your changing size. If you add a few items like these to your wardrobe, you can even share them with older or younger siblings.

■ It can be expensive to get clothes to fit your new shape. Instead of buying them new, check out second-hand clothing stores or trade clothes with friends.

You're Still You!

Although you may feel a little awkward around others at first, don't let the changes in your appearance make you withdraw from the world. Remember: *you're still you inside!* The qualities that other people like and admire in you—your friendliness, your sense of humor, your talents—don't go away!

Keeping Busy

TV, video games, and crossword puzzles can get old. Think you've run out of **things to do** while in the hospital or stuck at home? Think again! Here are 25 ideas sure to make **time fly!**

 1 "I painted my windows with pictures of everyone in my family. I felt happy whenever I looked at them. One day when I was feeling sick, I painted a sad face. It made me feel better to get out of bed and do something."

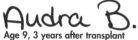
Age 9, 3 years after transplant

2 Tape-record a letter to your class at school, your best friend, or siblings at home.

3 Make a snack and watch videos of your family.

4 Organize a drawing contest for the kids on your unit. If you're in isolation, ask a nurse to announce the theme, such as the ultimate cake, athletic shoe, or evening gown. Then ask the nurse to collect the drawings, and pass them around for everyone to see and vote on. The most creative ideas win!

5 Imagine a dream vacation, sporting event, or concert you'd like to go to or participate in. Draw your ideas, write them down, or simply escape to these places in your mind whenever you want.

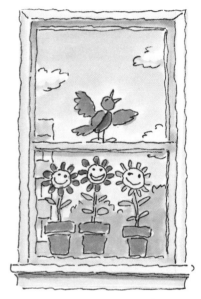

Turn your windows into works of art with washable paint. Design them to look like stained glass or paint a portrait of a precious pet.

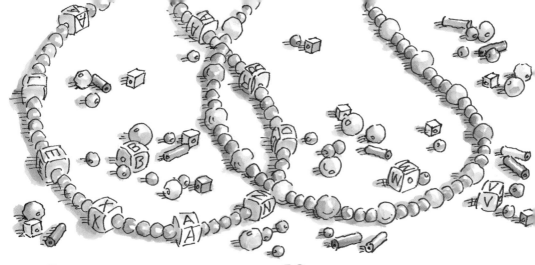

6 Make friendship bracelets with string and beads and hand them out to other kids on the unit.

7 & 8 "My aunt gave me a magic set, and I learned to do tricks. The doctors and nurses would ask for a new trick every day.

"I also play the piano, so I brought a keyboard to the hospital. The doctors would ask if I could learn certain songs to play for them. Making people around me happy made me feel happy in return."

Zachary Z.

Age 15, 5 years after transplant

10 Start a scrapbook or photo album or add to one you already have.

11 Make a cheer-up chart. Write down at least one good thing that happens to you each each day. Some days it may be as silly as "At least an elephant didn't sit on me today!"

12 Talk to new patients and try to help them out. Fill them in on your hospital and the staff.

13 Write a fan letter to your favorite singer, actor, athlete, or artist. Or if you've met kids you admire who've been through a transplant, drop them a line.

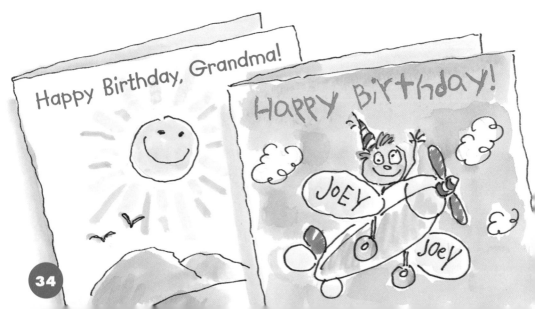

14 Start a mini-paper for your transplant unit. Interview other kids on the floor or ask them to submit short write-ups about themselves or stories they've written for fun. Arrange the "articles" so that they fit on just a few sheets of paper and glue them down, or use a computer if you have access to one. Add illustrations if you like, then photocopy your newspaper and hand it out.

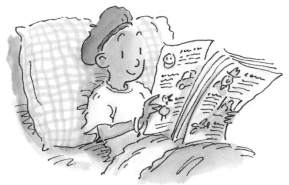

15 "When I got home from the hospital I started making a favorite craft again. I attach silk flowers to the tops of pens and put them in clay pots that I paint. My mom noticed that syringe caps were the perfect size to hold a pen upright, so we glue the caps in the pot and surround them with paper grass. We started selling the pens to stores and donate a portion of the money

 we make to the Leukemia Society. So far we've donated $200!

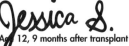
Jessica S.
Age 12, 9 months after transplant

16 Start a collection. Stamps, pencils, stickers, or postcards are some ideas. Let your friends and family know about your collection and invite them to help you add to it, but challenge them to do it by spending one dollar or less.

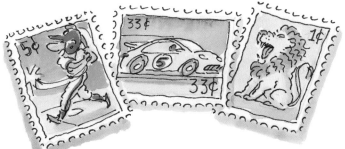

Cristina's Story

A Bright Idea

Cristina liked to keep busy during her 6-week stay in the hospital—it helped pass the time more quickly. When her nurses asked her to make decorations for the hallways, she gladly agreed. "First they asked me to do something to go with spring, so I drew bunnies and colored eggs. Later they wanted something summery," so Cristina drew lots of smiling suns. Even though she couldn't go out in the halls, the hospital staff and visitors were cheered by Cris-tina's art work—and that cheered Cristina!

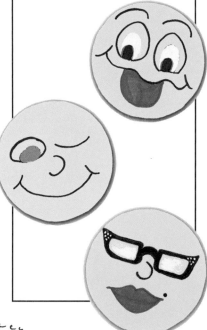

17 Sketch things or people in your room.

18 Start a diary or journal or add to one you already have. Here's one quick writing idea: using only 3 words, describe your day, the weather, a person, or your mood.

19 & 20 "I got a computer hook-up to my classroom while in the hospital. So that we always had something fun to talk about, I asked a new question every day, like: 'Today is National Eat Whatever You Want Day. What would you like to eat?'

"We also made a video for my class so they'd know what I was going through. They

 videotaped parties that I couldn't go to and sent me the tapes."

Robbie P.
Age 11, 7 weeks after transplant

21 If your friends can't visit, suggest that they get together at one friend's house and take turns talking on the telephone with you. If your hospital has provided your family with a video phone, maybe your friends can meet at your house and call you from there.

22 Compose a poem or song inspired by a powerful emotion you're feeling today.

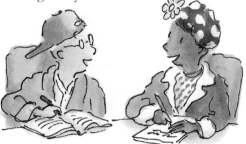

23 Catch up on your schoolwork. Learning is your job. You have a future to prepare for, so don't fall behind! Push yourself so that when you go back to school, you'll be on target. If your transplant center has a hospital school, try attending, or form study groups with other kids in your unit.

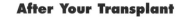

"One friend who wrote me said that we should start a story and send it back and forth, each adding a paragraph," Cristina says. "I always looked forward to getting mail from her because it was a fun activity."

24 & 25 "My mom painted pictures on my fingernails. I had mice, bears, flowers, and different-colored ying-yang symbols.

"She also brought in Easter decorations, and we decorated my room. We even dyed eggs and had an egg hunt!"

Jenny H.

Age 13, 1 1/2 years after transplant

Leaving the Hospital

The day you're finally able to leave the hospital may be filled with mixed emotions. You've probably **waited** for this event for weeks but now may be a little **nervous.** You might suddenly worry whether you are ready to be out on your own. It's a big step, but your doctors are letting you take it because they're **confident** you're **healthy** enough to go. Be proud of yourself—you've reached a major milestone!

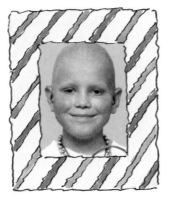

" My goal was to get out of the hospital so I could go see *Star Wars: Episode I* when it first came out. I still had to wait a week after I got home, wear a mask, and go when the theater wasn't as crowded, but it was great!"

chris S.
Age 10, 1 month after transplant

Stepping Out

If you'll be staying in the hospital for a long time, you may be allowed to take short trips away during the day before you're actually discharged. You'll probably have to wear a mask for protection and may even need to bring along your IV pole. The sights, sounds, and smells outside the hospital may be startling at first, especially if it's been a while since you've experienced them. These trips can also be exhausting, but they're great practice for when you go home for good.

Rules for Release

Hospitals have different rules for when transplant patients can be discharged to go home. Your white blood cell count will need to be high enough so that your body can begin to defend itself against everyday germs. The doctors and nurses will probably want you to be off antibiotics for a few days, and have had no fevers, nausea, vomiting, or diarrhea for several days in a row. If you're having trouble taking your medications by mouth, doctors may delay your discharge.

"I wanted to leave the hospital, but I was also kind of nervous." says Cristina. "I thought that I'd get sick again and would have to go back to stay for a longer time."

Clinic Visits

Even after your discharge, your recovery is not yet complete—your bone marrow is still not ready to meet the requirements of daily life. You'll have to make frequent trips back to your hospital's transplant clinic so doctors can examine you and treat any problems that may arise. (If you live far from your hospital, you'll probably stay in a nearby hotel or Ronald McDonald House before going home so you can return to the clinic easily. After a few weeks, you'll be able to go to a clinic closer to your house.)

At first, you'll have to visit the clinic daily or every other day. The time between your visits will gradually increase. Eventually you'll have checkups just once or twice a month, then once or twice a year. Occasionally patients need to return to the hospital for short stays if serious problems develop.

Healing at Home

Once you're home, it may take several months before you're ready to return to normal activities. Keep reaching for your goals, but also give yourself time to heal. At first you'll have to avoid crowded indoor places like malls, movie theaters, and churches or synagogues. You may be able to visit these places when fewer people are there—weekday mornings instead of weekend afternoons, for example. Your restrictions may be different than those of other kids who had their transplant the same time as you. You're recovering at different rates—try to be patient.

For a while, you'll probably have lots of medications to take. To keep track of them, make a chart showing how much of each you need and what time you should take it. It's important not to miss a dose—your recovery depends on it!

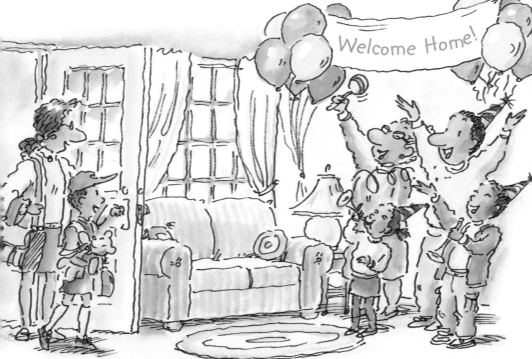

Eats and Treats

Your diet is an important part of your recovery. The right kinds of foods can help you stay **strong** and **heal** faster. Getting enough **nutrients** is also important because kids your age are often going through a growth spurt. If the side effects of your treatment have caused your appetite to shrink, try these 10 **taste-tempting** tips.

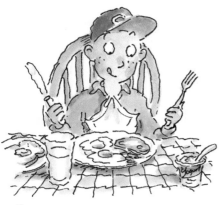

1 Eat whenever you're **hungry**—even if it's not mealtime. If a certain meal, like breakfast, appeals to you more than others, make it the largest meal of the day.

2 Eat even if you *don't* feel like eating, and even if you're on IV nutrition. Your stomach may have shrunk during your transplant. You need to stretch it out and **teach your body** to eat again.

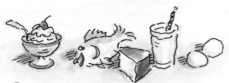

3 When you *do* eat, pick **protein**-rich foods like cheese, yogurt, fish, and eggs, which help the body repair itself. To keep your weight up, choose foods and drinks high in **calories**. (Give nutritional supplement shakes like Ensure a try.)

4 On days when you have a larger appetite, eat more to make up for days you ate less.

5 Vary what you eat. Try new foods and recipes—things you never liked before may taste good now. Ask your dietician for a list of good foods and recipes to try.

6 When you don't have an appetite for solid foods, try cool liquids. Your body needs water to function properly, so drinking fluids like shakes, fruit juices, sports drinks, or popsicles will help your body get the water it needs. Here's a delicious, nutritious shake to try:

Berry Fluff

- 1/2 cup frozen yogurt, berry-flavored
- 2 ounces cranberry juice
- 1 tablespoon wheat germ

Combine ingredients and blend.

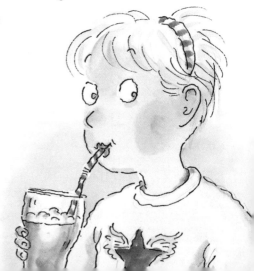

7 Eat **snacks** anytime. A few bites or sips of high-calorie foods or liquids every hour will keep your calorie intake up. Snacks can also surprise you by making you want to eat more. Try these tasty treats: cheese and crackers, chocolate milk, muffins, cereal, and pizza. Here's another super snack to sample:

Peanut-Butter Balls

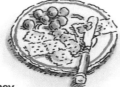

- 1 teaspoon vanilla extract
- 1 tablespoon nonfat instant dry milk
- 1 teaspoon water
- 1 teaspoon pasteurized honey
- 5 tablespoons peanut butter from a freshly opened jar Mix first 3 ingredients together. Then add honey and peanut butter, stirring slowly. Form into balls and chill as candy snacks or spread on crackers as snackers.

8 Experiment with eating in **different places.** A meal may taste better if served as a picnic on the patio or your family room floor.

9 **Exercise** an hour before mealtime—it may help make you more hungry. (Check with your doctor to make sure he or she approves.)

10 Boost a food's calorie or protein content with tasty **add-ins.** Here are some to try:

Adding Calories

Granola (without dried fruit):
Sprinkle on ice cream or oatmeal. Add to cookie or muffin batters.
Ice cream/frozen yogurt: Sandwich between cake slices or cookies. Blend with fruit juices or soda.
Honey or jam: Drizzle on cereal, toast, or shakes.
Butter: Add to noodles, rice, and sandwiches.
Whipped cream: Use on hot cocoa and desserts.

Adding Protein

Peanut butter:
Spread on muffins, waffles, or pancakes. Swirl through milkshakes or ice cream.
Cheese: Melt on hot dogs, hamburgers, sandwiches, or tortillas. Grate into soups, mashed potatoes, and vegetables.
Meats: Wrap in pie crust or biscuit dough to make a turnover. Sprinkle into soups, omelettes, or baked potatoes.

Food for Thought

Keep these points in mind when it's eating time:

✔ Think before you drink — don't share straws or eat off someone else's fork or spoon.

✔ If food that might be touched by others is passed at a meal, take your portion first.

✔ As food is being prepared, anyone tasting it should use a separate, clean spoon.

✔ All foods must be well cooked. No cold cuts, salads, or fresh (or dried) fruits or vegetables.

✔ Foods prepackaged in individual serving sizes are ideal!

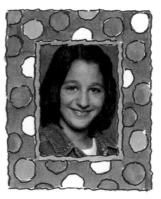

"All of a sudden I wanted to try things I'd never eaten before—like an olive loaf I saw in the store one day. I usually wanted spicier foods than I ate before."

Brittany P.
Age 12, 3 years after transplant

Family Matters!

Your whole family had to **adjust** to you being away at the hospital, and maybe a parent being there with you. If you were gone for a while, it may take time—and **patience**—to get used to being together again. The good news is, many kids say their transplant brought them **closer** to their family. These pages can help you do the same.

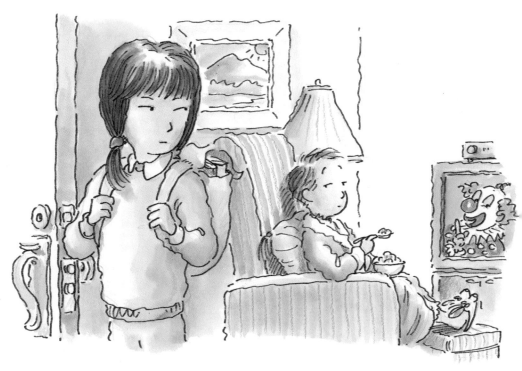

Sibling Struggles

Brothers and sisters can sometimes be jealous of the attention you get, even if they understand why you're getting it. They may also be upset that you get special privileges like different things to eat or not going to school. At the same time, they might feel guilty that they're well and can do fun things while you're stuck at home. All of these emotions may make them unsure about how to act. They might be extra-nice or get upset for silly reasons. These tips may help smooth the stormy times:

■ Show family members you appreciate them with smiles, hugs, and kind words. Play games with brothers and sisters or offer to help them with schoolwork.

■ If a sibling's actions are bothering you, explain how you feel without getting angry and let your sibling do the same. Then each should listen calmly to what the other has to say.

Parent Problems

Your transplant has been difficult for your parents. They've watched you endure painful procedures and may have felt unable to comfort you. Now that you're home, they may be extra-cautious about your health—you might think they're over-protective. Moms or dads may also fight more due to stress or being overly tired themselves. As you recover, they'll start to relax and get better, too. Here are some other things you can do to relieve the tension:

■ **Do your part to care for yourself. Take your medicine and eat when you can to take strain off your parents.**

■ **It's important to tell parents about your aches, ills, or extreme fatigue. So that they don't overreact, be specific when describing your symptoms. For example, try to recognize whether you're *really* tired or just very bored.**

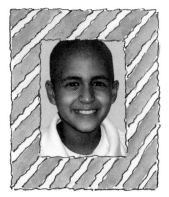

"Some medicines make me crabby—I don't want to talk or have anybody talk to me. I tell people when I feel that way so they'll come back at a better time."

Jacob R.
Age 10, 1 month after transplant

Getting Along Again

There may be days when you realize you're the one overreacting or lashing out at family unfairly.

■ **Remember, medications may cause moodiness.**

■ **It's also common to feel angry at people who are well. You may be taking your frustrations out on others because you're anxious to get better. If you *do* blow up, try to calm down before the argument gets out of hand. Take time to cool off; then apologize if you've said things you're sorry about.**

Sometimes good things can come out of bad. The rough times your family may be going through can actually improve your relationships. As you try to understand each other's feelings and talk through your problems, you may all grow closer.

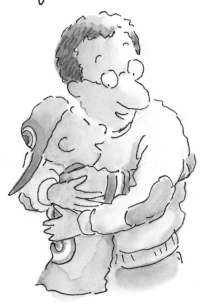

"My siblings either didn't talk to me or they babied me," Cristina says. "When they were *too* nice, I wanted them to act more like normal. But now I wish it was back to that," she laughs.

Back to School

Easing into It

Your doctor will let you know when you can return to school. If you received your own marrow or stem cells, you may be able to go back 3 to 6 months after your transplant. Otherwise, it may be a year before you can return. Until you do, a tutor can help you at home. If classmates can sometimes bring you schoolwork, it'll help you stay in touch while you're away.

When you *are* ready to return to class, you may start out going a few hours a day, and as you feel stronger, work your way up to full-time. Your parents should let your teachers know that you may need to have snacks or rest periods during the day, take medications, or use the bathroom more often.

Fitting in Again

Returning to school can be exciting, but you may also worry that classmates will treat you differently. It can take a little time for things to feel normal again. If you look different—have lost hair or weight or are wearing a mask—some kids might avoid you because they don't know what to say or how to act. They may need you to break the ice. First, make sure you haven't withdrawn from them out of embarrassment or fear of what they might think—classmates might mistake your nervousness as being unfriendly. It may also help to explain your transplant to them and answer questions they may be curious about.

Talking about your transplant can clear up misunderstandings classmates may have.

Friends Forever?

If you've been away for a while, it might seem as if some friends have moved on to new interests or friendships while you were gone. Don't assume this is so—give yourselves a chance to get comfortable with one another again. Sometimes friends are worried that things will change between you, when they just want everything to be the same. Reassure them that you're still the same person. Once they realize this, they'll usually relax and treat you like before. Some kids say they make new friends after their transplant, and that their new friends are better buddies than they had before.

What to Say

You may wonder what you'll say about your changed appearance to friends or others who are curious. Try explaining it straight out: "The medicine I'm taking for my transplant makes my face bloated, but I'll return to normal after I stop taking it." Some kids say using humor helps put classmates more at ease. If you've met other kids who have been through a transplant, you might ask what approaches worked for them.

Keeping Up

Chemotherapy and radiation therapy can sometimes affect your memory, handwriting, or ability to concentrate or organize things. Some kids say math is more difficult for them since their transplant. You and your parents should meet with your teachers to set up study goals. When you reach your goals, you'll feel good about yourself and your schoolwork.

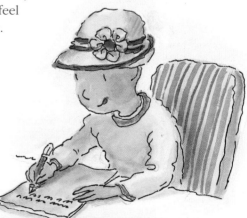

Focus on the Future

For many transplant patients, it takes a year or more to **recover** both **physically** and **emotionally** following their transplant. Even after a year is up, your life may not completely return to the way it was before. Here are some **issues** you may be dealing with.

Late Effects

Some complications don't develop until months or even years after a transplant.

Inability to fight infections: It can take a year or two for your marrow's infection-fighting system to fully recover. Some patients continue to experience serious infections until then.

Chronic GVHD: GVHD that appears after Day 100 is called "chronic." You can develop chronic even if you never had "acute." (Remember, if you received your own cells, GVHD won't occur.) Symptoms of chronic are: skin that thickens or darkens; stiff joints; muscle shrinkage; jaundice; dry, burning eyes; and mouth sores. To treat chronic GVHD, you need to return to infection-prevention routines and go back on drugs to keep your new marrow from attacking your body organs.

Growth problems: Many kids who had radiation therapy experience some delay in growth. You may be given growth hormones, which can sometimes help you catch up.

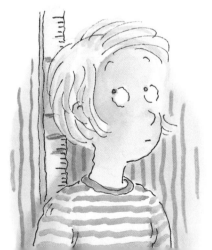

Dental problems: If you didn't have your adult teeth before your transplant, their development may be delayed due to radiation therapy. Tooth decay and gum disease are also common, so see a dentist regularly and don't forget good oral hygiene!

Cataracts: Cataracts are cloudy spots on the eyes that blur vision. They can result from radiation therapy and develop 3 to 6 years after a BMT. If you notice a change in the way you see, tell a parent. Cataracts can be removed to restore your eyesight.

Relapse: The return of your original disease is called "relapse." It's common for patients to worry that they're having a relapse whenever they feel a little sick. As time passes, though, you'll worry less. With each year you remain healthy, your chances of being cured for good are better and better.

A+ Attitude

Lasting problems can be frustrating. If you *are* experiencing one or more of these late effects, try to focus on what you *can* control—such as mouth care, nutrition, and exercise—and leave other worries to your doctors.

There may also be days you feel so good you're tempted to skip your check-up. Remember: it's important to go! If complications *are* starting to form, doctors need to treat them while they're small to keep them from getting worse.

How You've Changed

Kids who have been through a bone marrow transplant often think they look at life differently afterwards. Many feel they make the most of each day now and don't waste time being unhappy about unimportant things. Others say the experience made them mentally stronger and able to handle tough situations. If a problem arises, they have more confidence they can overcome it.

What's your outlook on life now? Can you see how you may have benefited by your transplant experience? Did you develop or discover personal traits that you're proud of? We hope so! To learn how you can share your new insights and experiences with others, turn the page.

Your transplant experience might make you want to develop new talents or try things you've never tried before.

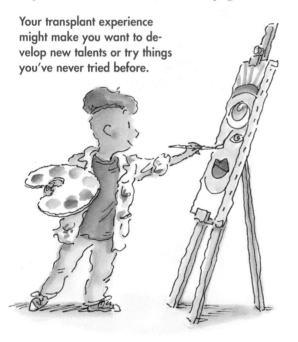

turn the page.

Bouncing Back

If you just haven't felt like your normal self since your transplant, try getting involved in activities that help you feel good about your skills.

Some kids take dancing lessons or a martial art like karate or judo to improve their concentration and coordination. Others discover that playing their favorite sport helps restore their strength and self-confidence. A new hobby like painting or playing a musical instrument can help you develop new interests and pride.

Just don't forget: as a transplant survivor, you already have a lot to be proud of!

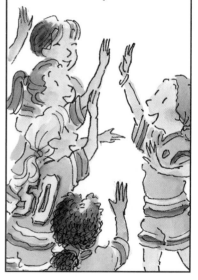

"I love my life now!" Cristina says. "I used to be afraid of what other people thought of me. Now I realize that life is short, so you have to live it fully and do what you feel—don't let anybody stop you."

Get Better, Give Back!

Where Is She Now?

These days, Cristina's favorite activities include cheerleading and acting and singing in plays. "The cheerleading gives me a lot of exercise and it's really fun," she says, "but I *love* being up on stage singing in front of everybody. Before I had the BMT, I would have been shaking. Now I'm not even nervous!"

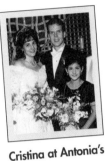

Cristina at Antonia's wedding

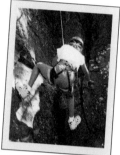

Cristina rock climbing

Cristina also finds great satisfaction in visiting other kids who are going through BMTs. "Every Christmas since I got well, we go to the hospital and give out little gifts like fun pencils, word searches, decks of cards, and little games," Cristina says. "I like seeing kids smile. They just look so much happier afterwards. It makes *me* feel better, too!"

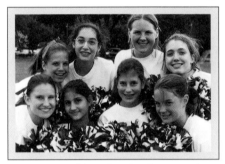

Cristina and her cheerleading squad

What You Can Do

Would you like to help out other kids the way the kids in this book helped you? Here are some suggestions for sharing your time and talents:

■ Start a pen-pal program at your school. Each of your classmates can write to a different transplant patient.

■ Organize a toy collection for the kids at the nearest transplant center.

■ Write cards or make decorations to send to transplant patients at holiday time.

■ Attend or volunteer to be a counselor at a summer camp where you'll meet other kids who are former transplant patients.

■ Hold a fundraiser in your town to benefit transplant patients.

■ Visit our website at: http://www.astellas.us/pncr/books.php or write to the address below and tell us about your transplant experience. We'll post as many comments as we can on this site so that other kids can learn from you what to expect. Let us hear from you!

Astellas Pharma US, Inc.
Medical Information Dept.
Parkway North Center
Three Parkway North
Deerfield, IL 60015-2548